Essential Lists
for Intercollegiate
MRCS

Essential Lists for Intercollegiate MRCS

Michael O. Murphy MRCS
Department of Vascular Surgery
Manchester Royal Infirmary
Manchester

Edited by

James Hill FRCS ChM
Consultant General Surgeon
Manchester Royal Infirmary
Manchester

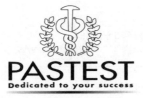

PASTEST
Dedicated to your success

© 2004 PasTest Ltd
Egerton Court
Parkgate Estate
Knutsford
Cheshire, WA16 8DX

Telephone: 01565 752000

First edition 2004

ISBN: 1 901198 23 5

A catalogue record for this book is available from the British Library.

The information contained within this book was obtained by the authors
from reliable sources. However, while every effort has been made to ensure
its accuracy, no responsibility for loss, damage or injury occasioned to any
person acting or refraining from action as a result of information contained
herein can be accepted by the publisher or the authors.

PasTest Revision Books and Intensive Courses

PasTest has been established in the field of postgraduate medical education
since 1972, providing revision books and intensive study courses for doctors
preparing for their professional examinations. Books and courses are
available for the following specialties:

**MRCP Part 1 and Part 2, MRCPCH Part 1 and Part 2, MRCOG, DRCOG,
MRCGP, MRCPsych, DCH, FRCA, MRCS and PLAB.**

For further details contact:

PasTest Ltd, Freepost, Knutsford, Cheshire, WA16 7BR
**Tel: 01565 752000   Fax: 01565 650264
Email: enquiries@pastest.co.uk   Web site: www. pastest.co.uk**

Typeset by Vision Typesetting Ltd, Manchester
Printed and bound in Europe by the Alden Group

Contents

For my mother and father for reminding me
what it is all about.

Michael Murphy is a research fellow and MD student at the Department of Vascular Surgery, Manchester Royal Infirmary.

Foreword

Knowledge may be at the bottom of the pyramid of learning, but it forms the foundations for competence and performance. As such, assessment of knowledge is an important part of postgraduate surgical examinations. The new curricula in general surgery are identifying for trainees what needs to be learned and at what stage in their training.

This book, written by a trainee who has recently overcome the MRCS hurdle, is also intended to make life a little easier for those soon to take the 'test'.

The classifications, definitions, causes and associations included in this text are based on the MRCS curriculum and common topics in the examination. The reader should use it as a source of facts and an aide-memoire.

JH   May 2004

Glossary

↑	increased
↓	decreased
1°	primary
2°	secondary
#	fracture
AAA	abdominal aortic aneurysm
Ab	antibody
ABO	ABO blood group system
ACE	angiotensin-converting enzyme
AD	autosomal dominant
ADH	antidiuretic hormone
AF	atrial fibrillation
AFP	α-fetoprotein
Ag	antigen
ALI	acute lung injury
Ant.	anterior
AP	abdomino-perineal
AR	autosomal recessive
ARDS	acute respiratory distress syndrome
Art.	artery
ASA	American Society of Anesthesiology
ATN	acute tubular necrosis
AT III	antithrombin III
A-V	arteriovenous

AVM	arteriovenous malformation
AVN	avascular necrosis
BCC	basal cell carcinoma
BP	blood pressure
BZD	benzodiazepines
CA	carcinoma
Cap	capillary
CCF	congestive cardiac failure
CEA	carcinoembryonic antigen
CF	cystic fibrosis
Chol	cholesterol
CJD	Creutzfeldt–Jakob disease
CML	chronic myeloid leukaemia
CMV	cytomegalovirus
CNS	central nervous system
CO	carbon monoxide
Col.	colloid
COPD	chronic obstructive pulmonary disease
CRC	colorectal cancer
CRH	corticotropic releasing hormone
CRP	C reactive protein
Cry.	crystalloid
CVA	cerebrovascular accident
CVP	central venous pressure
DIC	disseminated intravascular coagulation
DM	diabetes mellitus
DNA	deoxyribonucleic acid
DPG	diphosphoglycerol
DPL	diagnostic peritoneal lavage
DVT	deep venous thrombosis
dx	disease
EBV	Epstein–Barr virus
ECG	electrocardiogram
EMD	electromechanical disassociation

EN	enteral nutrition
ENT	ear nose and throat
ERCP	endoscopic retrograde cholangiopancreatography
ESR	erythrocyte sedimentation rate
FAP	familial adenomatous polyposis
G6PD	glucose-6-phosphate dehydrogenase
GCS	Glasgow coma scale
GH	growth hormone
GIT	gastrointestinal tract
GN	glomerulonephritis
GU	genitourinary
HbF	fetal haemoglobin
βhCG	beta human chorionic gonadotrophin
Hep	hepatitis
HHV	human herpesvirus
HIV	human immunodeficiency virus
HNPCC	hereditary non-polyposis colon cancer
HPOA	hypertrophic pulmonary osteoarthropathy
HPV	human papilloma virus
HTLV	human T-lymphotropic virus
Hx	history
IBD	inflammatory bowel disease
ICP	intracranial pressure
Ig	immunoglobulin
IHD	ischaemic heart disease
ITP	idiopathic thrombocytopenia purpura
ITU	intensive care unit
IVC	inferior vena cava
JVP	jugular venous pressure
LA	left atrium
LFT	liver function test
LIF	left iliac fossa
LN	lymphadenopathy
LVF	left ventricular failure

MEN	multiple endocrine neoplasia
Met.	Metastasis
MI	myocardial infarction
MND	motor neurone disease
MODS	multiorgan dysfunction syndrome
MS	multiple sclerosis
(N)	normal
NFM	neurofibromatosis
NG	nasogastric
NJ	nasojejunal
NSAID	non-steroidal anti-inflammatory drug
NSCLC	non-small cell lung cancer
NYHA	New York heart association
OA	osteoarthritis
OCP	oral contraceptive pill
P2	pulmonary heart sound
p_aO_2	partial pressure of oxygen
paeds.	paediatrics
PAN	polyarteritis nodosum
PAWP	pulmonary artery wedge pressure
PE	pulmonary embolus
PEG	percutaneous endoscopic gastrostomy
PICC	peripherally inserted central catheter
PK	pyruvate kinase
PPP	pancreatic polypeptide
PR	per rectum
PRV	polycythaemia rubra vera
PSA	prostate specific antigen
PT	prothrombin time
RA	rheumatoid arthritis
RCC	red cell count
RIF	right iliac fossa
RNA	ribonucleic acid
RSD	reflex sympathetic dystrophy

RUQ	right upper quadrant
RVF	right ventricular failure
SCC	squamous cell carcinoma
SCLC	small cell lung cancer
SFJ	saphenofemoral junction
SIADH	syndrome of inappropriate anti-diuretic hormone
SIRS	systemic inflammatory response syndrome
SLE	systemic lupus erythematosis
Staph.	staphylococci
Strep	streptococci
Sx	surgery
Syn.	syndrome
TB	tuberculosis
Temp.	temperature
TG	triglyceride
TIA	transient ischaemic attack
TIPS	transjugular intrahepatic porto-systemic shunt
TPN	total parenteral nutrition
TPR	total peripheral resistance
TR	tricuspid regurgitation
TRALI	transfusion related acute lung injury
TSH	thyroid stimulating hormone
TUR	transuretheral resection
TURP	transuretheral resection of the prostate
UMN	upper motor neurone
UTI	urinary tract infection
UV	ultraviolet
VIP	vasoactive intestinal peptide
Vol.	volume
WCC	white cell count
ZN	zinc

CHAPTER ONE

Anaesthetics and ITU

Anaesthetics and ITU

SYSTEMIC INFLAMMATORY RESPONSE SYNDROME (SIRS)

(Harmful and excessive response to an insult in the acute phase)

Two or more of the following:
Tachycardia   > 90 beats minute^{-1}
Tachypnoea   > 20 breaths minute^{-1}
Temperature < 36 °C or > 38° C
WCC   > 12 or < 4 × 10^3/mm

CAUSES OF ACUTE RESPIRATORY DISTRESS SYNDROME (ARDS)

(Refractory hypoxia in appropriate clinical setting with bilateral diffuse pulmonary infiltrates and a PAWP < 18 mmHg and P_aO_2/FIO_2 < 200)

Direct:
Aspiration
Pulmonary contusion
Toxic gas inhalation
Near drowning
Pneumonia
Fat embolus
Radiation

Indirect:
Sepsis
DIC
Trauma
Cardiopulmonary bypass
Blood transfusion
Pancreatitis
Reperfusion injury
Burns

3

NYHA ASSESSMENT OF CARDIOVASCULAR FUNCTION

I   no limitation of ordinary physical activity
II   slight limitation of ordinary physical activity or ordinary activity result in palpitations, dyspnoea or angina
III   marked limitation of physical activity. Less than ordinary activity results in palpitations, dyspnoea or angina
IV   inability to carry out any physical activity without discomfort which may occur at rest

ASA GRADING (+E for Emergency)

I   healthy individual
II   mild systemic disease
III   severe systemic disease that limits activity but is not incapacitating
IV   incapacitating disease that is a constant threat to life
V   moribund – not expected to survive with or without an operation

POST MI RISK OF RE-INFARCTION PERI-OPERATIVELY

<3 weeks	80%
3 weeks – 3 months	20–30%
3–6 months	5–15%
>6 months	1–4%
Peri-operative MI mortality	50%

(Baseline peri-operative MI rate is 0.2% of which half are silent and most are on the third post-operative day)

BENEFITS OF EPIDURAL POST OP

Improved respiratory function
↓ Diaphragmatic splinting
↓ DVT
↓ Urinary retention
Earlier mobilisation

↓ Sympathetic stimulation
↓ Cardiac workload
↓ Vascular resistance
↑ Splanchnic blood flow

ENDOCRINE RESPONSE TO STRESS/SURGERY

Catecholamines (adrenal medulla):	Inotropic and chronotropic Lipolysis Gluconeogenesis
Cortisol (adrenal cortex):	Proteolysis Lipolysis Gluconeogenesis
Aldosterone (adrenal cortex):	Na^+ and water retention
ADH (posterior pituitary):	Water retention
GH (anterior pituitary):	Gluconeogenesis Insulin resistance
Glucagon (pancreatic G cells):	Glycogenolysis Gluconeogenesis ↓ Insulin secretion

SUXAMETHONIUM SIDE EFFECTS

Muscle pain	Hyperkalaemia
Bradycardia	Hypo/hypertension
Bronchospasm	Malignant hyperpyrexia

COMPLICATIONS OF GENERAL ANAESTHESIA

Aspiration	Atelectasis
↑ Sputum production	Segmental collapse (V/Q mismatching)
↓ Cough reflexes	↑ CO_2
↓ Ciliary activity	ARDS

COMPLICATIONS OF VENTILATION

Barotrauma (pneumomediastinum/thorax, subcutaneous emphysema)
Volutrauma
Air embolism
↓ Cardiac output
Nosocomial pneumonia
Parenchymal lung damage

COMPLICATIONS OF INTUBATION

Trauma to teeth or upper airway
Procedural hypoxia
Aspiration
Haemorrhage

Blockage
Misplacement
Cuff puncture/displacement

INDICATIONS FOR INTUBATION

↓ GCS/impaired gag reflex
High risk of airway obstruction
Airway protection
Bronchial toilet

Hypoxia
Metabolic acidosis
CO_2 retention
To counteract ↑ ICP

PROBLEMS WITH PULSE OXIMETRY

Measures oxygenation not ventilation
Inaccurate at O_2 saturation < 90%
Read out is 2–3 seconds behind real time
Interference from abnormal haemoglobin:

CO poisoning
Bilirubin

Smokers
Methaemoglobin

Interference with signal:

Shivering
Bright light

Diathermy
Nail varnish

Interference with flow:

Hypotension
Vasoconstriction

Hypovolaemia

SHIFTS O_2/SATURATION CURVE RIGHT (decreases affinity of Hb for p_aO_2

↓ p_aO_2
↑ H^+
↑ 2,3 DPG

Pyrexia
Haemoglobin F (fetal)
Altitude

RESPIRATORY FAILURE

Type I: $p_aO_2 < 8$ kPa and $p_aCO_2 < 6.7$ kPa)

Acute asthma	ARDS
COPD/emphysema	PE
Pneumonia	Pulmonary fibrosis
Atelectasis	Haemo/pneumothorax

Type II: $p_aO_2 < 8$ kPa and $p_aCO_2 < 6.7$ kPa)

Severe asthma	Spinal injury
Severe COPD/emphysema	Head injury
Bronchiectasis	↑ ICP
Kyphoscoliosis	Coma
Chest wall trauma	Opioids
Abdominal distension	Muscular dystrophy
Phrenic nerve injury	Myasthenia gravis
Sleep apnoea	Guillian–Barré syndrome

ACID BASE DISORDERS

Respiratory acidosis:	Respiratory alkalosis:
CVA	CVA
CNS tumour	PE
Encephalitis	Encephalitis
Sedation/opioids	Hypoxia in COPD
↑ ICP	Hyperventilation/panic attack
Neuromuscular disease	Exercise
Trauma/surgery	Altitude
Ankylosing spondylitis	Salicyclate (early in poisoning)
COPD	Amphetamine
Pneumonia	Pulmonary oedema

Metabolic acidosis:	Metabolic alkalosis:
Ketoacidosis	Vomiting
Acute renal failure	Chronic renal failure
Lactic acidosis (see below)	Hyperaldosteronism
Methanol/ethanol	Iatrogenic, eg diuretics
Fistulae/diarrhoea	Alkali abuse
TPN	
Salicylate (late in poisoning)	

CAUSES OF LACTIC ACIDOSIS

Shock (see below)
Pancreatitis
Liver impairment/failure
Renal impairment/failure
Excessive exercise
Leukaemia
Biguanides

POST OP HYPOXIA

Pneumonia   Opioids
Atelectasis   ARDS/ALI
Bronchospasm   PE
Pneumothorax   Pulmonary oedema
Diaphragmatic splinting Tracheal compression
Poor analgesia

IV FLUIDS

Crystalloids:

	Na^+ mmol/l	Cl^- mmol/l	Dextrose g/l	K^+ mmol/l	Osmolality mosm/l
Normal saline	154	154	0	0	308
Dextrose	0	0	50	0	252
1/5 Normal saline	30	30	40	0	286
Hartmann's	131	111	0	5	279
Ringers lactate	147	156	0	4	273

Colloids:
  Albumin
  Gelofusine
  Dextrans (40,70)
  Penta/Hetastarch

TYPES OF SHOCK

	Temp.	CVP	BP	TPR
Hypovolaemic	↓/–	↓	↓	↑
Septic	↑/↓	↓	↓	↓
Cardiogenic	↓/–	↑	↓	↑
Anaphylactic	↑/–	↓	↓	↓
Neurogenic	–	↓	↓	↓

CLASSES OF SHOCK

Class	I	II
Vol loss	10–15% (0.75 L)	30–40% (1.5 L)
Pulse rate	<100	>100
BP	–	–
Pulse pressure	–	↓
Urine output	>30	>20
Resp rate	<20	<30
Consciousness	Restless	Anxious
Fluid	Crystalloid	Cry/colloid
Skin	Normal	Clammy

Class	III	IV
Vol loss	30–40% (<2 L)	>40% (>2 L)
Pulse rate	120	>140
BP	↓	↓
Pulse pressure	↓	↓
Urine output	>5	0
Resp rate	<40	>40
Consciousness	Confused	Lethargic/coma
Fluid	Colloid/blood	Colloid/blood
Skin	↓Cap. refill	Pale/cold

INDICATIONS FOR SWAN GANZ CATHETER (ie CVP ≠ LA pressure)

Valvular heart disease
LVF and interstitial pulmonary oedema
Chronic severe lung disease
Assessing hemodynamic response to therapies
Diagnosis and assessment of pulmonary hypertension
Diagnosis and assessment of shock states
Diagnosis and assessment of ARDS/MODS
Instability after cardiac surgery

CAUSES OF RAISED CVP

CCF   Tension pneumothorax
MI with RVF   Pericardial effusion
Overload   Cardiac tamponade
Cardiac contusion   TR
SVC obstruction

FEATURES OF TENSION PNEUMOTHORAX

Respiratory distress   Tracheal deviation away from side
↑ JVP   Ipsilateral decreased breath sounds
EMD arrest   Ipsilateral hyper-resonance

FEATURES OF CARDIAC TAMPONADE

↑ JVP
Muffled heart sounds
↓ BP
Kussmaul's sign
EMD arrest
(First three are known as Beck's triad)

CARDIAC SUPPORT (INOTROPES)

	α_1	α_2	β_1	β_2	D_1	D_2
Dopamine	++	+	++	++	+++	++
Dobutamine	–	–	+++	+	–	–
Adrenaline	++	++	+++	+++	–	–
Noradrenaline	+++	++	+++	+	–	–
Isoprenaline	–	–	+++	+++	–	–

INDICATIONS FOR RENAL REPLACEMENT THERAPY IN RENAL FAILURE

Persistent hyperkalaemia – > 6.0
Acidosis pH – < 7.2
Pulmonary oedema
Fluid overload despite diuresis
Drug clearance, eg sedatives
Uraemic complications, eg pericarditis, tamponade

RENAL FAILURE

Pre-renal: Hypovolaemic shock   Renal artery trauma/embolus
             Septic shock   Renal artery stenosis
             Cardiogenic shock   Compartment/crush syndrome
             Anaphylactic shock

Renal: ATN   Vasculitis
             Hypertension   Interstitial nephritis
             Diabetic disease   Goodpasture's syndrome
             Glomerulonephritis   Renal vein thrombosis/embolism
             Infection/pyelonephritis

Post-renal: Bladder outlet obstruction Stricture
             Stones   Retroperitoneal fibrosis
             Blocked catheter   Neoplasm
             Infection

CHILD'S CLASSIFICATION OF SEVERITY IN CHRONIC LIVER DISEASE

	1	2	3
Bilirubin (μmol/l)	<35	35–50	>50
Albumin (g/l)	>35	30–35	<30
Ascites	None	Mild	Marked
Encephalopathy	None	Mild	Advanced
Nutrition/prothrombin time (seconds prolonged)	Good/ >4 s	Moderate/ 4–6 s	Poor/ >6 s

* Patient is grouped from A to C where A is <7, B 7–9 and C >9

(Original classification used nutrition but later modified to prothrombin time increase)

SURGICAL PROBLEMS ASSOCIATED WITH OBESITY

DM	More wound infections
IHD	↑ DVT/PE
Atelectasis	↑ Dissection/tissue trauma
↑ Risk of aspiration	Longer duration of surgery
Difficult intubation	Larger wounds

FEED TYPES

Enteral (EN):	Oral
	NG
	PEG
	NJ
	Jejunostomy
Parenteral (TPN):	Peripheral line
	PICC
	Central line

ADVANTAGES OF EN OVER TPN

Cheaper
Increased gut blood flow
Decreased gut translocation
Decreased stress ulceration
Maintains gall bladder function
More effective energy usage by portal system
Fewer infections
Less line associated complications

FUNCTIONS OF ELEMENTS IN FEEDS

Vitamin A – epithelial cell proliferation and differentiation
Vitamin B_6 – collagen cross-linkage
Vitamin C – collagen cross-linkage and transport
Vitamin D – calcium and phosphate metabolism
Carbohydrate – prevents ketosis during a stress response
Proteins – extracellular matrix
Zinc – RNA/DNA synthesis, metalloproteases, antibacterial
Copper – collagen and elastin cross-linkage
Selenium – anti-oxidant

COMPLICATIONS OF EN

Tube related:	Misplacement	Leakage
	Displacement	Blockage
Feed related:	Diarrhoea	Nausea/vomiting
	Bloating/colic	Drug interactions
	Refeeding syndrome	

COMPLICATIONS OF TPN

Line related: Sepsis/infective endocarditis   Thoracic duct injury
Thrombophlebitis   Chylothorax
Pneumothorax   Embolism
Haemothorax   Lost guide wire
Nerve injury   Arrhythmia
Vascular injury/haematoma   Perforated right atrium

Feed related: $\uparrow \downarrow$ Glucose, Na^+, K^+, H^+ Fatty liver
$\uparrow$ Ca^{++}, CL^- Abnormal LFTs
$\downarrow$ Folate, Zn, PO_4^-, Mg^{++} Gall bladder stasis
Fluid overload   Refeeding syndrome

STEROID EQUIVALENCE

Hydrocortisone	20 mg	Triamcinalone	4 mg
Prednisolone	5 mg	Betamethasone	0.75 mg
Methylprednisolone	4 mg	Dexamethasone	0.75 mg

TRANSPLANT REJECTIONS

Hyperacute – preformed antibody (hours)
Accelerated acute – secondary antibody response (days)
Acute – cytotoxic T-cell mediated (weeks)
Chronic – antibody-mediated vascular damage (months – controversial)

AUTOIMMUNE DISEASE

Hashimoto's thyroiditis – Thyroglobulin + microsome
Graves' disease – TSH receptor
Atrophic gastritis – Parietal cells
Pernicious anaemia – Intrinsic factor
Goodpasture's syndrome – Basement membrane
Myasthenia Gravis – Acetylcholine receptor
Systemic Lupus erythematosis – DNA smooth muscle
Rheumatoid Arthritis – IgM
Scleroderma – Centromere

Primary biliary cirrhosis – Mitochondria
Insulin-dependent DM – Pancreatic islet cells
Guillian–Barré syndrome – Peripheral nerve myelin

CAUSES OF IMMUNOSUPPRESSION

Congenital:
   Agammaglobulinaemia
   Hypogammaglobulinaemia
   IgA deficiency
   Common variable immunodeficiency
   Selective antibody deficiency

Acquired:
   Infectious – HIV, systemic infection
   Iatrogenic – Splenectomy, transfusion, radiotherapy, chemotherapy, steroids
   Neoplastic – Leukaemia, lymphoma, myeloproliferative diseases, advanced solid tumours
   Other – Hypoxia, DM, alcoholism, poor nutrition, trauma/surgery

CAUSES OF POST-OPERATIVE PYREXIA

Physiological response
Drug-induced
DVT/PE
Anastomotic leak
Abscess

Respiratory tract infection
Urinary tract infection
Wound infection
Cannula site infection

RISK FACTORS FOR WOUND INFECTION

Operative factors:
   Emergency surgery
   Extended pre-op admission
   Site of incision, eg peri-anal
   Excessive tension
   Poor tissue handling

   Pre-op shaving
   Necrotic tissue
   Tissue ischaemia
   Faecal peritonitis
   Intra-abdominal abscess

Patient factors:

Extremes of age	Immunosuppression (see above)
Poor nutritional status	Cardiac failure
Obesity	Renal failure
DM	Hepatic failure
Alcoholism	Respiratory failure

ANTIBIOTICS

Bacteriocidal: β-lactams
                 Aminoglycosides
                 Vancomycin
                 Chloramphenicol

Bacteriostatic: Tetracycline
                 Erythromycin
                 Clindamycin

STERILISATION (kills everything including viruses and spores)

Autoclave	Dry heat
Ethylene oxide	Low temperature steam with formaldehyde
Irradiation	

DISINFECTION (kills everything except some viruses and spores)

Boiling water	Iodophors/iodine
Low temperature steam	Alcohol
Formaldehyde	Hydrogen peroxide

NORMAL COMMENSAL ORGANISMS

Skin –   staph, strep, corynebacteria, Propionibacter
Nasal – staph
Oral –   staph, strep, *Neisseria*, *Haemophilus*, corynebacteria, anaerobes

Upper GIT – staph, strep, *Neisseria*, *Haemophilus*, corynebacteria, clostridium, yeasts
Lower GIT – Enterobacteriaceae, enterococci, bacteroides, clostridium, yeasts
GU – Enterobacteriaceae, enterococci, bacteroides, clostridium, yeasts, staph, strep, lactobacilli, corynebacteria

CLASSIFICATION OF WOUND

Clean – uninflammed tissue with no GU/GI tract entry (<2% infection rate)
Clean-contaminated – entry to hollow viscus other than colon with minimal contamination. (8–10% infection rate)
Contaminated – spillage from hollow viscus, eg colon, open fractures or bites (12–20% infection rate)
Dirty – frank pus, perforated viscus, traumatic wound (>25% infection rate)

TUMOURS IN HIV

Lymphoma – non-Hodgkin's lymphoma
Squamous cell carcinoma – skin, cervix, larynx
Kaposi's sarcoma
Squamous cell papilloma

ACUTE ABDOMEN IN HIV

Bacterial enteritis
Megacolon 2° to CMV
Haemorrhage 2° to GI involvement by Kaposi's sarcoma, lymphoma
Pancreatitis 2° to anti-retroviral therapy
Tuberculous disease of the GI tract
Normal surgical disease in HIV +ve patient

TOXINS

	Exotoxin	Endotoxin
Bacteria	Gram +ve and –ve	Gram –ve
Source	Intracellular	Cell wall
Structure	Polypeptide	Lipopolysaccharide
Effect	Variable	Septic shock
Vaccine	Yes	No
Heat stable	No	Yes

CHAPTER TWO

General Surgery and Urology

General Surgery and Urology

CAUSES OF ANYTHING (SURGICAL SIEVE)

Congenital

Acquired
Infective	Degenerative
Inflammatory	Endocrine/metabolic
Immunological	Neoplastic
Iatrogenic	Traumatic
Vascular	Psychogenic

COMPLICATIONS OF DIATHERMY

Explosion – alcohol, bowel obstruction
Electrocution – patient, surgeon
Burn – skin, inflammable spirit
Channelling – penis, digit
Coupling – especially in laparoscopic surgery
Interference – pacemaker

FUNCTIONS OF THE PERITONEUM

Allows movement of the viscera
Suspends viscera
Conveys vessels, lymphatics and nerves
Stores fat
Absorbs contaminants
Seals off infected/ulcerated surfaces

LUMPS

Site
Size
Shape
Surface
Scar
Skin change
Surround (edge)

Temperature
Tenderness
Transilluminance
Thrill/bruit
Compressibility
Colour
Consistency

Fixity (superficial and deep)
Fluctuance
Expansile/pulsatile
Associated LN
Reducibility

CAUSES OF CLUBBING

GI:	Coeliac disease	Cirrhosis
	IBD	GI lymphoma
Lung:	Lung CA	Empyema
	Fibrosing alveolitis	Bronchiectasis/CF
	Mesothelioma	
Cardiac:	Cyanotic heart disease	Atrial myxoma
	Infective endocarditis	
Other:	Familial	Axillary aneurysm
	Graves' acropathy	Brachial A-V malformation

SKIN ULCERS

Edge:	Sloping (healing)	Punched out (ischaemic/
	Rolled (BCC)	neuropathic)
	Everted (SCC)	Undermined (necrotic/TB)
Base:	Granulated	Malignant
	Slough	
Floor:	Fascia	Bone
	Muscle	
Discharge:	Serous	Purulent
	Sanguineous	

GRANULOMATOUS DISEASES

TB (caseating)
Fungal infections
Helminth infections
Langerhan's histiocytosis
Malignancy
Churg–Strauss syndrome
Sarcoidosis
Wegener's granulomatosis
Hypersensitivity

GYNAECOLOGICAL CAUSES OF ABDOMINAL PAIN

Ruptured ectopic pregnancy
Endometriosis
Torsion/rupture of ovarian cyst
Uterine fibroids
Mittelschmerz
Pelvic inflammatory disease
Adenomycosis
Tubo-ovarian abscess

NEONATAL CAUSES OF ABDOMINAL PAIN

Malrotation
Meconium plug/Ileus
Hirschsprung's disease
Necrotising enterocolitis
GIT stenosis
GIT atresia
Diaphragmatic hernia
Gastroschisis/Exomphalos

PAEDIATRIC PYLORIC STENOSIS

Projectile non-bilious vomiting
Hungry post vomiting
Dehydration
Weight loss
Olive-shaped mass in RUQ
Visible peristalsis
Metabolic alkalosis
Hypokalaemic hypochloraemia

INTUSSUSCEPTION

Pallor
Childhood colic/irritability
Normal between attacks
Bilious vomiting
Red current jelly stool/PR bleed
Distension
Dehydration

GI PROBLEMS IN ALCOHOL ABUSE

Gastritis
Gastric ulceration
Acute pancreatitis
Chronic pancreatitis
Pancreatic cancer

Oesophageal SCC
Portal hypertension
Hepatocellular carcinoma
Liver cirrhosis
Fatty liver/hepatitis

RETROPERITONEAL FIBROSIS

Aortic aneurysm
Radiation
Lymphoma
Idiopathic
Methysergide

REFERRED PAIN

Ruptured liver – R shoulder tip
Ruptured spleen – L shoulder tip
Gall bladder – between scapulae/R shoulder
Pancreatitis/AAA – back
Ureteric colic – ispilateral groin/genitalia
Testicular pain – ispilateral flank
Abdominal surgery – both shoulder tips

HODGKIN'S DISEASE

Lymphocyte proliferative (10%) prognosis good
Nodular sclerosing (65%)   prognosis good
Mixed cellularity (20%)   prognosis moderate
Lymphocyte depleted (5%)   prognosis poor

POSITIVE DIAGNOSTIC PERITONEAL LAVAGE
(false +ve 15%/ false –ve 2%)

> 100 000 RCC/mm^3
> 500 WBC/mm^3
DPL fluid in chest drain/urinary catheter
Bowel contents on DPL
Gram stain +ve

DIAPHRAGMATIC OPENINGS

T12 – aorta, azygos, thoracic duct
T10 – oesophagus, L and R vagus nerve
T8 – IVC, R phrenic nerve
Medial arcuate ligament – sympathetic trunk
Lateral arcuate ligament – subcostal artery and nerve
Posterior xiphoid – superior epigastric vessels
Posterior hernia – foramen of Bochdalek
Anterior hernia – foramen of Morgagni

PRESENTATION OF LUNG CA

Locoregional disease:	Cough	Chest pain
	Haemoptysis	Pneumonia
	Horner's syndrome	Hoarseness
	LN	
Secondary disease:	Bone pain	Jaundice
General symptoms:	Anorexia	Weight loss
Paraneoplastic:	ACTH excess	Clubbing (HPOA)
	SIADH	Neurological

CAUSES OF PLEURAL EFFUSION

Transudate:	Cardiac failure	Hypoproteinaemia
	Liver failure	Protein losing enteropathy
	Renal failure	Hypothyroidism

Exudate: Lung CA   Pneumonia
                Lung metastases   TB
                Mesothelioma   Lung abscess
                Lymphoma   Subphrenic abscess
                Asbestosis   RA/SLE/vasculitis
                Pancreatitis   Dressler's syndrome
                Chylothorax   Meig's syndrome
                PE

BODY FLUID CONSTITUENTS

	Volume	Na^+	K^+	HCO_3^-	Cl^-
Saliva	0.5–1.5L	30	20	40	15
Stomach	1.5–2.5L	60	10	0	150
Duodenum	1.5L	140	5	25	100
Pancreas	0.5–1.5L	140	5	100	70
Bile	0.5–1.0L	140	5	40	100
Jejunum and ileum	2.5–3.5L	140	5	25	100
Colon	0.5L	70	20	0	50
Sweat	0.5–2.0L	50	10	0	50

SUTURES

Absorbable:

Vicryl	Polyglactin	Synthetic	Braided
PDS	Polydiaxonone	Synthetic	Monofilament
Maxon	Polyglyconate	Synthetic	Monofilament
Dexon	Polyglycolic acid	Synthetic	Braided
Catgut	Bovine intestine	Natural	Monofilament

Non-absorbable:

Prolene	Polypropylene	Synthetic	Monofilament
Steel	Steel	Synthetic	Monofilament
Ticron	Polyester	Synthetic	Braided
Ethilon	Nylon	Synthetic	Monofilament
Silk	Silkworm	Natural	Braided

ESSENTIAL CRITERIA FOR SCREENING

Related to disease:	Serious	Latent
	Important	Common
	Treatable	Outcome affected by earlier detection
Related to test:	Sensitive	Acceptable
	Specific	Cheap
	Safe	

TUMOUR MARKERS

PSA – prostate
CEA – colon
AFP – gonadal/liver
Thyroglobulin – thyroid
Calcitonin – medullary cell CA

βhCG – gonadal/choriocarcinoma
CA125 – gonadal
CA153 – metastatic disease
CA19.9 – pancreatic

CANCERS THAT METASTASISE TO

Liver:	GI	Lung
	Pancreas	Breast
	Urological	Melanoma
Lung:	Kidney	Colorectal
	Germ cell	Breast
	Sarcoma	Melanoma
Bone:	Lung	Kidney
	Breast	Thyroid
	Prostate	
Brain:	Lung	Melanoma
	Kidney	Colon
	Breast	
Adrenal:	Lung	Breast

CARCINOGENS

Chemical: β Naphthalene – bladder
Aflatoxin – liver
Asbestos – lung and mesothelial surfaces
Benzopyrene – lung
Chromium/nickel/arsenic – lung
Nitrates – stomach

Infective: Schistosomiasis – bladder
Hep B+C – liver
EBV – nasopharyngeal/Burkitt's lymphoma
HPV – cervical and anal
HTLV 1 – leukaemia
HHV 8 – Karposi's sarcoma

Radiation: UV – skin
Ionising – leukaemia, bone, breast, thyroid, skin, ENT

PROTO-ONCOGENES AND MALIGNANCY

Nuclear:	MYC	Burkitt's lymphoma
	n-MYC	Neuroblastoma
	l-MYC	SCLC
Transduction:	RAS	Lung, colon, pancreatic
	Ab1	Acute lymphoid leukaemia
Growth factor:	SIS	Astrocytoma
	hst-1	Osteosarcoma
	int-2	Stomach, bladder, breast
Growth factor inhibitor:	Erb B1	Glioma
	Erb B2	Breast, ovary, stomach
	Ret	Medullary CA of thyroid
Tumour suppressor:	p53	Many
	E-cadherin	Stomach
	APC	Colon
	DCC	Stomach, colon, pancreas
	NF1+2	NFM, Schwannoma, sarcoma
	Rb	Retinoblastoma, osteosarcoma
	Wt-1	Wilm's tumour

| RNA repair genes: | Msh-2 | HNPCC |
| Apoptosis: | Bcl-2 | B cell lymphoma |

ABNORMALITIES OF GROWTH

Hyperplasia   Hamartoma
Hypertrophy   Teratoma
Metaplasia   Neoplasia
Dysplasia

COMPLICATIONS OF RADIOTHERAPY

Early: Fatigue/malaise   Bleeding
            Nausea/vomiting   Erythema
            Diarrhoea   Ulceration
            Desquamation   Oesophagitis
            Bone marrow suppression

Late: Pneumonitis   Infertility
            Pulmonary fibrosis   Early menopause
            IHD   Cataracts
            Bowel strictures   2° malignancies
            Adhesion   Renal failure
            Bladder fibrosis   Delayed wound healing
            Hypothyroidism   Lymphoedema

CAUSES OF DYSPHAGIA

Neurological: CVA   Achalasia
                MND   Chagas' Dx
                MS   Nutcracker oesophagus
                Parkinson's Dx   Diffuse oesophageal spasm
                Muscular dystrophy

Mechanical: Pharyngeal pouch   Goitre
                Oropharyngeal tumour   Stomach CA
                Tonsillitis   Lung CA
                Oesophageal CA   Thoracic aneurysm
                Oesophageal web   Post op stricture
                Oesophageal bar/ring

CAUSES OF UPPER GI BLEEDING

Duodenal ulcer/erosion   Mallory Weiss tear
Gastric ulcer/erosion   Angiodysplasia
Oesophageal ulcer/erosion   Hereditary haemorrhagic telangiectasia
Upper GI malignancy   Dieulafoy's lesion
Varices

RISK FACTORS FOR GASTRIC CA

Dietary – nitrates, salt, vitamin deficiency A, C, E
H. pylori
Pernicious anaemia
Previous gastric surgery
Family history of gastric CA
Gastritis/ulceration/polyps
ABO group A (diffuse rather than intestinal type)
Japanese
Male

ALARM SYMPTOMS IN UPPER GI MALIGNANCY

Persistent dyspepsia > 45 years   Unintentional weight loss
Dysphagia/odynophagia   Previous gastric surgery
Persistent vomiting   Previous gastric ulcer
Iron-deficiency anaemia   Suspicious barium meal
GI bleed   Epigastric mass
NSAID use   Epigastric pain requiring
                                    hospitalisation

LATE COMPLICATIONS OF GASTRIC SURGERY

Diarrhoea   Dumping (early and late)
Biliary reflux   Anaemia (B_{12}, Fe^{++}, folate deficiency)
Malnutrition   Bezoar
Malignancy   Gastric outlet obstruction
Early satiety   Gall stones

COMPLICATIONS OF STOMAS

Local: Ischaemia/necrosis   Spillage to efferent loop
          Prolapse   Leakage
          Retraction   Skin excoriation
          Stenosis   Haemorrhage
          Parastomal hernia   Flatus/odour
          Intussusception   Granulomata

Systemic: Nutritional disorders   Diarrhoea
          Kidney stones   Psychological/sexual
          Gall stones   Social
          Short gut syndrome

DIFFERENTIATING STOMAS

	Ileostomy	Colostomy
Site	RIF	LIF
Surface	Spout	Flush
Content	Watery	Containing faeces
Permanent	Panproctocolectomy	AP resection
Temporary	Loop ileostomy	Hartmann's
	(Ant resection)	

PARALYTIC ILEUS

Local: Post-operative   Retroperitoneal haematoma
            Peritonitis   Mesenteric ischaemia/infarction
            Abscess   Abdominal trauma
            Pancreatitis

Systemic: Pneumonia   Uraemia
            Spinal injury   Ketoacidosis
            Hypercalcaemia   Burns
            Hypokalaemia   Sepsis
            Jaundice   Opioids

INTESTINAL FISTULA

Anastomotic leakage
Diverticular disease
Crohn's disease
Carcinoma
Post-operative
Radiation
Embryological
Traumatic

OBSTRUCTION

Functional:

Paralytic ileus
Pseudo-obstruction

Mechanical small bowel:

Luminal – gallstone ileus, helminths, bezoar
Mural – Crohn's, TB, malignancy, radiation
Extraluminal – adhesions, hernia, volvulus

Mechanical large bowel:

Luminal – constipation
Mural – colorectal CA, diverticular disease,
         Crohn's disease, ischaemic stricture
Extraluminal – volvulus

ASSOCIATED WITH FAP

Dental cysts
Retinal pigmentation
Duodenal adenomas/CA
Jaw osteomas
Colorectal polyps/CA
Epidermoid cysts
Abdominal desmoid tumours
Hamartomatous polyps of the stomach

AMSTERDAM CRITERIA – HNPCC

$\geq$ 3 family members with CRC
CRC in $\geq$ 2 generations
$\geq$ 1 first-degree relative
$\geq$ 1 at less than 45 years of age
FAP excluded

DUKE'S CLASSIFICATION AND SURVIVAL

		Rectal (%)	Colon (%)
A	Confined to wall	90	90
B	Through the wall but LN −ve	65	65
C_1	LN +ve but not the apical node	40	35
C_2	LN +ve and the apical node	25	–
D	Metastasis	15	<5

Originally for rectal CA with no C_2 or D stages

RISK FACTORS FOR COLORECTAL CANCER

Inflammatory bowel disease >10 years
Ureterosigmoidostomy
Gastric surgery
Low fibre diet
HNPCC
FAP incl Gardener's syndrome
Turcot's syndrome
Canada–Cronkhite syndrome

FEATURES OF COLORECTAL CA

Change in bowel habit
PR bleeding/mucus
Tenesmus
Fistula
Rectal mass
Iron-deficiency anaemia
Abdominal distension/obstruction
Abdominal mass
Perforation

DISTRIBUTION OF COLORECTAL CANCER

Rectal	35%	Descending	10%
Sigmoid	25%	Transverse	10%
Caecal	15%	Ascending	5%

EXTRA-INTESTINAL FEATURES OF IBD

Related to disease activity: Pyoderma gangrenosum
                               Erythema nodosum
                               Aphthous ulcer
                               Arthropathy/arthritis

Unrelated to disease activity: Sacroilitis/ankylosing spondylitis
                               Fatty liver/cirrhosis
                               Chronic active hepatitis
                               Primary sclerosing cholangitis
                               Cholangiocarcinoma/hepatoma
                               Gall stones/kidney stones
                               Amyloidosis
                               Clubbing
                               Conjunctivitis/uveitis/episcleritis

ASSOCIATED WITH PYODERMA GANGRENOSUM

Ulcerative colitis   PRV
Crohn's disease   Myeloma
PAN   Autoimmune hepatitis
Idiopathic   Leukaemia
IgA paraproteinaemia   SLE/RA

BARIUM ENEMA FEATURES OF IBD

Crohn's disease: Skip lesions   Rosethorn ulcers
                   Fistulae   Cobblestoning
                   Strictures   String sign

Ulcerative colitis: Pseudopolyps   Hose piping
                    Loss of haustrae Shortened colon
                    Ulceration

INDICATIONS FOR SURGERY IN IBD

Toxic megacolon

Perforation

Malignant transformation

Bleeding

Recurrent exacerbations

Stricture

Intra-abdominal abscess

Intestinal fistulae

Peri-anal sepsis

Failure to thrive in children

Failed medical treatment

COMPLICATIONS OF DIVERTICULAR DISEASE

Phlegmon

Abscess

Fistula

Perforation

Bleeding

Benign stricture

LOWER GI BLEEDING

Diverticular disease

Angiodysplasia/A-V malformation

Colorectal carcinoma

Haemorrhoids

Inflammatory bowel disease

Hereditary telangiectasia

Radiation proctitis

Ischaemic colitis

Drugs – NSAIDS, warfarin

Infective colitis

Meckel's diverticulum

Adenomatous polyps

Anal fissure/rectal ulcer

Haemangioma

Wegener's granulomatosis

Rheumatoid arthritis

Endometriosis

Juvenile polyps/intussusception (paeds)

MECKEL'S DIVERTICULUM

Twice as common in males

Asymptomatic before 2 years

2 cm long

2 feet proximal to ileocaecal valve

2 types of tissue (gastric and pancreatic)

2% of the population

CAUSES OF CIRRHOSIS

Cryptogenic (30%)
Alcohol (25%)
Chronic active hepatitis (Hep B+C)
Autoimmune hepatitis
Drugs, eg methotrexate, isoniazid
Wilson's disease
Haemochromatosis
Post-hepatic obstruction (see below)
Hepatic vein obstruction

Primary biliary cirrhosis
Secondary hepatic fibrosis
Sarcoidosis
α_1 Anti-trypsin deficiency
Galactosaemia
Glycogen storage diseases
Vitamin A toxicity
CF

CAUSES OF HEPATOMEGALY

Infective:
Hepatitis B+C
EBV
CMV
TB
Weil's disease

Liver abscess
Malaria
Hydatid disease
Schistosomiasis

Obstructive:
Gall stones
Stricture

Pancreatic cancer
Acute/chronic pancreatitis

Depositional:
Wilson's
Haemachromatosis

Amyloid
Fatty liver

Congestive:
CCF/TR

Budd–Chiari syndrome

Other:
Cirrhosis
COPD
Liver CA/metastases
Lymphoma

Reidel's lobe
Reticulosis
Liver cysts
Lympho/myeloproliferative dx

RISK FACTORS FOR HEPATOCELLULAR CARCINOMA

Cirrhosis (see above)
Hepatitis B + C
Aflatoxin (*Aspergillus flavus*)
α_1 Anti-trypsin deficiency

CAUSES OF ASCITES

↑Portal venous pressure:	Portal vein thrombosis	Budd–Chiari syndrome
	Lymphadenopathy	Constrictive pericarditis
	Cirrhosis	CCF/TR
	Metastasis	Pulmonary hypertension

Hypoproteinaemia:	Renal failure	Cachexia
	Liver failure	Protein losing enteropathy
	Cardiac failure	

Peritonitis:	Post-irradiation	Carcinomatosis
	Bacterial peritonitis	Pseudomyxoma
	Tuberculous peritonitis	Uraemia
	Pancreatitis	Talc granulomas

Chylous:	Trauma	Congenital abnormality
	Lymphatic disease	Thoracic duct obstruction

Endocrine:	Hyperaldosteronism	Hypothyroidism

CAUSES OF JAUNDICE

Pre-hepatic:	Haemolysis	Sepsis
	CCF	

Congenital:	Crigler–Najjar syndrome	Rotor's syndrome
	Dubin–Johnson syndrome	Gilbert's disease

Hepatic:	Alcohol	Haemachromatosis
	Cryptogenic	Wilson's disease
	Liver metastasis	Primary biliary cirrhosis
	Hepatocellular CA	Glycogen storage disease
	CCF/TR	Galactosaemia
	Budd-Chiari syndrome	α_1-anti-trypsin deficiency
	Physiological (neonates)	SLE/scleroderma
	Pregnancy	Cystic fibrosis

Infective:	Hep A-E	Malaria
	EBV	Schistosomiasis
	CMV	Amoebiasis
	HIV	Toxoplasmosis

Drugs:	Halothane	Isoniazid/rifampicin
	Paracetamol	Valproate
	Co-amoxiclav	Chlorpromazine
	Erythromycin	Methyldopa
	OCP	Methotrexate
	Tamoxifen	Barbituates

Post-hepatic:	Pancreatic CA	Gall stones
	Cholangio CA	Primary sclerosing cholangitis
	Hepatocellular CA	Stricture
	Gall bladder CA	Choledochal cyst
	Hilar lymphadenopathy	Mirizzi's syndrome
	Acute/chronic pancreatitis	

CAUSES OF PORTAL HYPERTENSION

Pre-hepatic:	Portal/splenic vein thrombosis	Splenomegaly
	A-V fistula	Tumour
	Congenital malformation	

Hepatic:	Cirrhosis (see above)	Polycystic disease
	Schistosomiasis	

Post-hepatic:	Budd–Chiari syndrome	Hepatic vein invasion
	Veno–occlusive disease	Constrictive pericarditis
	Caval obstruction	CCF/TR

INDICATIONS FOR TIPS

Uncontrolled acute variceal haemorrhage
Failed endoscopic treatment
Awaiting liver transplant
Not fit for surgery

COMPLICATIONS OF VARICEAL HAEMORRHAGES

Aspiration
Pneumonia
Hypoxia
Renal failure
Hepatic encephalopathy
Exsanguination

CAUSES OF SPLENOMEGALY

Bacterial –	typhoid, TB, septicaemia, leptospirosis, syphilis, brucella
Viral –	hep A-E, EBV, CMV, HIV
Protozoan –	malaria, kala azar, hydatid disease
Deposition –	amyloid, Gaucher's dx, Felty's dx, Still's dx, sarcoid
Congestion –	CCF, hepatic vein obstruction, portal hypertension, cirrhosis
Haematological –	leukaemia, lymphoma, pernicious anaemia, PRV, elliptocytosis, spherocytosis, ITP, sickle cell disease
Infarction –	bacterial endocarditis, atrial fibrillation, mural thrombus post-MI
Solitary –	cystic disease, lymphosarcoma, angioma

FUNCTIONS OF SPLEEN

Immunological –	produce IgM, capture foreign antigens
Filtration –	encapsulated bacteria
Sequestration –	old erythrocytes and platelets
Storage –	platelets (30%), iron
Haematopoiesis –	embryological, haemolytic anaemia

INDICATIONS FOR SPLENECTOMY

Trauma	Hodgkin's disease
Immune – ITP, haemolytic anaemia	Hairy cell leukaemia/CML
Congenital – elliptosis, spherocytosis	Part of solid tumour resection
Splenic vein thrombosis	Thalassaemia
Gaucher's disease	Splenic abscess/cyst
Myelofibrosis	

CAUSES OF ACUTE PANCREATITIS

Gall stones
Alcohol
Idiopathic
Trauma
Pancreatic CA
Iatrogenic – ERCP, post-op., radiation
Drugs – Diuretics, steroids, chemotherapy
Metabolic – ↑ Ca^{++}, ↑ TG, ↑ cortisol, ↓ temp
Infective – CMV, mumps, coxsackie
Congenital – CF, haemochromatosis, cystic disease, pancreas divisum

LUMP IN GROIN/ILIAC FOSSA

Inguinal hernia
Femoral hernia
Obturator hernia
Transplanted kidney
Ectopic testis
Sebaceous cyst
Lipoma
TB ileum
Appendix mass/abscess

Saphena varix
Femoral artery aneurysm
Enlarged LN
Sarcoma
Psoas abscess
Psoas bursitis
Caecal CA
Bladder diverticulum

UMBILICAL HERNIA

3% of live births
Operate at ≥ 3 years old
0.3% need repair
Recurs in 3rd trimester
Most regress by age 2

CONTENTS OF INGUINAL CANAL

Artery to the vas
Testicular artery
Cremasteric artery

Ilioinguinal nerve
Genital nerve
Sympathetic nerve

Vas/round ligament
Pampiniform plexus
Lymphatics

PRE-DISPOSING FACTORS FOR UTI

Urinary obstruction
Diabetes
Pregnancy
Congenital anomalies
Female

Instrumentation/catheterisation
Extremes of age
Calculi
Constipation

RENAL STONES

Calcium oxalate (74%)
Calcium phosphate (8%)
Struvite (MAG 9%)
Urate (7%)

Cysteine (1%)
Xanthine (<1%)
Silicate (<1%)
Matrix (<1%)

COMPLICATIONS OF CALCULI

Obstruction
Stricture
Infection
Malignant change

Haemorrhage
Perforation
Metaplasia

ENLARGED KIDNEY

Hydronephrosis
Solitary cysts
Polycystic kidneys
Renal cell CA
Hypertrophy of single kidney
Horseshoe kidney

Peri-nephric abscess
Pyonephrosis
Renal vein thrombosis
DM
Amyloidosis
SLE

COMPLICATIONS OF TURP

Immediate: Haemorrhage
             Sepsis
             TUR syndrome (1%)

Early: Secondary haemorrhage
             Sepsis
             Clot retention (1%)

Late: Stricture
             Incontinence (1%)
             Erectile dysfunction (20%)
             Retrograde ejaculation (70%)

TYPES OF HYDROCOELE

Vaginal (testes)
Hydrocoele of the cord (cord)
Congenital hydrocoele (communicates with peritoneum)
Infantile (cord and testes)
Secondary (tumour, torsion, trauma, orchitis, post-op)

INDICATIONS FOR CIRCUMCISION

Phimosis   Penile CA
Paraphimosis   Recurrent UTIs
Recurrent balanitis   Religious
Xerotica balanitis obliterans

COMMON CONGENITAL URINARY ABNORMALITIES

Horseshoe kidney
Pelvi–ureteric junction obstruction
Ureteric duplication
Vesico–ureteric junction obstruction
Ureterocele
Posterior urethral valves

CHAPTER THREE

Orthopaedics and Neurology

Orthopaedics and Neurology

STAGES OF FRACTURE HEALING

Immediate – tissue death and haematoma formation from torn blood vessels and AVN

Reactive – inflammation and cellular proliferation with bridging of fracture site. There is also angiogenesis with haematoma resorption

Regeneration – reaction of chondrocytes and osteocytes to form woven bone providing anchorage but with little tensile strength (callus)

Consolidation – appearance of osteoblasts and osteoclasts leading to lamellar bone formation

Remodelling – repair of site to normal bone density with improvement in alignment and strength, and restoration of medullary cavity

OSTEOPOROSIS

Primary: Post-menopausal
Idiopathic
Familial

Secondary: Endocrine – Addison's Dx, Cushing's Dx, hyperparathyroidism, thyroid Dx, DM, hypogonadism
Neoplasm – pituitary tumour, myeloma, carcinomatosis
Drugs – steroids, heparin, chemotherapy, antiepileptics
Dietary – vitamin C + D deficiency, malnutrition, alcoholism, malabsorbtion

45

COMPLICATIONS OF FRACTURES

	Local	General
Early:	Neurovascular injury	DIC
	Visceral injury	Hypovolaemic shock
	Haematoma	Crush injury
	Infection	Atelectasis
	Soft tissue swelling	SIRS
	Skin loss	Fat embolism
	Compartment syndrome	
Late:	Delayed union	DVT
	Malunion	PE
	Non-union	Urinary tract infection
	Joint stiffness	Respiratory tract infection
	OA of joint	Disuse atrophy
	Synostosis	Renal stones
	Subluxation/dislocation	Osteoporosis
	Skin necrosis	Psychological
	Pressure sore	Economic
	Contracture	
	Re-fracture	
	Avascular necrosis	
	Sudeck's atrophy/RSD	
	Myositis ossificans	
	Tendon rupture	
	Osteomyelitis	
	Pseudoaneurysm formation	

POOR HEALING IN BONE

Infection	Inadequate immobilisation
DM	Displacement
Poor blood supply	Dietary deficiency of Ca^{++}, PO_4^-, vitamin D
Comminuted fracture	

TYPES OF FRACTURE

Traumatic/Stress/Pathological
Incomplete/Complete/Greenstick
Open/Closed
Comminuted/Simple

TREATMENT OF FRACTURES

Reassure
Relieve pain
Reduce
Rehabilitate
Rigid (hold)

BLOOD LOSS WITH FRACTURES

Pelvis –   1–5L
Femur –   1–2.5L
Tibia –   0.5–1.5L
Humerus – 0.5–1.5L

INTERNAL VS EXTERNAL FIXATION

	Advantages	Disadvantages
Internal fixation:	Early mobilisation	Needs surgery
	Precise	Expensive
	↓ Pain	Soft tissue damage
		Infection
External fixation:	Simple	Cumbersome
	Safe	Pin tracking
	Fast	Infection
	Re-usable	Compliant patient
	Versatile	More aftercare
	Open fractures	

GUSTILO–ANDERSON CLASSIFICATION OF OPEN FRACTURE

I   wound < 1 cm, little soft tissue damage, minimal comminution, simple fracture
II wound > 1 cm, moderate soft tissue damage, moderate comminution, moderate contamination or a high energy injury
III extensive soft tissue injury, comminution or contamination
        + (a) inadequate soft tissue coverage, comminuted and segmental
        + (b) extensive soft tissue damage with massive contamination and contaminates requiring local/free flap
        + (c) arterial injury requiring repair

SALTER–HARRIS CLASSIFICATION

I   separation of epiphysis and metaphysis
II fracture of metaphysis
III fracture of epiphysis
IV fracture of epiphysis and metaphysis
V   crushing of growth plate

BONE TUMOURS

	Benign	Malignant
Bone	Osteoid osteoma (osteoma)	Osteosarcoma
	Osteoblastoma	–
Cartilage	Chondroblastoma	–
	Osteochondroma	Chondrosarcoma
Fibrous	Fibroma	Fibrosarcoma
	Fibrous dysplasia	–
Vessel	Angioma	Angiosarcoma
Marrow	–	Myeloma
	–	Ewing's sarcoma
Misc	Giant cell tumour	–
	Brown tumour	–

ARTHRITIDES

	Rheumatoid arthritis	Osteoarthritis
Worse	In the morning	At night
Relieved by	Exercise	Rest
Morning stiffness	> 30 minutes	< 30 minutes
Relieves	NSAIDs	Simple analgesia
History	Family history, Systemic effects	History of trauma Occupational
↑ESR / CRP	+	−
Anaemia	+	−
Synovial fluid	Inflammatory	Non-inflammatory
Extra-articular disease	Present in 20%	Absent
X-ray findings	Peri-articular Osteoporosis Joint space narrowing Subchondral cysts Erosions	Peri-articular Osteophytes Joint space narrowing Sclerosis
Clinical findings	Subluxation Soft tissue swelling Boutonniere deformity Swan sign Z deformity	Heberden's nodes Bouchard's nodes

EXTRA-ARTICULAR DISEASE IN RHEUMATOID ARTHRITIS

Eyes –   Sjörgen's syndrome, cataracts, episcleritis
Chest –   pericarditis, effusions, lung granuloma, fibrosing
               alveolitis, nodules, bronchiolitis obliterans
Autoimmune disease –   Graves' disease, Addison's disease, myasthenia
               gravis, vitiligo
General –   lymphadenopathy, splenomegaly (Felty's),
               carpal tunnel syndrome, vasculitis

DUPUYTREN'S CONTRACTURE

Familial (AD)
Idiopathic
Age
Occupational
Trauma
Cirrhosis
Alcohol
Smoking
DM
Phenytoin
Peyronie's disease
HIV

DUPUYTREN'S AFFECTS IN ORDER

Ring
Little
Middle
Index
Thumb

COLLES' FRACTURE

Pathological   Dorsal displacement
Within 2.5 cm of wrist   Radial displacement
Extra-articular   Dorsal angulation
Shortened   ± Fracture of ulnar styloid
Impacted

CLASSIFICATION OF ANKLE FRACTURE – WEBER

A   below syndesmosis (transverse)
B   at syndesmosis (spiral or oblique)
C   above syndesmosis (syndesmotic injury)

CLASSIFICATION OF HIP FRACTURE – GARDEN

I   impacted fracture that is undisplaced and incomplete (one cortex)
II   complete fracture that is undisplaced (both cortices)
III   complete fracture with partial displacement
IV   complete fracture with complete displacement

COMPLICATIONS OF TOTAL HIP REPLACEMENT

Perforation/fracture of acetabulum
Recurrent dislocation
Sciatic nerve injury
Loosening
Periprosthetic fracture
Leg length discrepancy

DVT
Infection
Fat embolus
Heterotopic calcification
Thigh pain
Gait problems

CAUSES OF LIMPING IN A CHILD

Irritable hip
Perthes' disease
Fracture
Slipped upper femoral epiphysis
Septic arthritis

GAIT TYPES

Antalgic:	Pain	↑ Swing phase
Trendelenberg:	Weak abductors	'Hip dip'
Parkinsonian:	Parkinson's disease	Shuffling/festinate
Broad based:	Cerebellar	Lurches to one side
Short leg:	Previous #, congenital	Hip drops

ORTHOPAEDICS AND NEUROLOGY

High stepping:	Foot drop	No heel strike
Spastic:	UMN lesion	Jerky
Waddling:	Proximal myopathy	Shifting from side to side

CAUSES OF LOCKED KNEE

Meniscal tear/discoid meniscus   Synovial chondromatosis
Cruciate ligament injury   Femoral condyle dysplasia (child)
Loose body   Osteochondritis desiccans (young adult)
Fracture   Intra-articular tumour (elderly)

TYPES OF INTRACRANIAL HAEMATOMA

Extradural – Direct trauma with # especially temporal and parietal lobes (arterial)
Intracerebral – Direct trauma or 2° to DM, hypertension or tumour
Subdural – Sheer force tears bridging veins (acute/chronic)
Subarachnoid – Arterial rupture from Berry aneurysm or AVM

SKULL FORAMINA

Rotundum – maxillary V_2
Ovale – mandibular V_3
Spinosum – meningeal art
Lacerum – internal carotid art
Superior Orbital Fissure – oculomotor III, trochlear IV, ophthalamic V_1, abducens VI
Jugular – accessory XI, vagus X, glossopharyngeal IX
Hypoglossal – hypoglossal XII
Magnum – spinal accessory XI
Optic canal – optic II, ophthalamic art

CEREBRAL LOBE FUNCTIONS

Frontal: Emotion
Personality
Speech (motor)
Motor

Parietal: Sensory
Spatial orientation
Speech (sensory)

Temporal: Memory
Smell

Occipital: Vision

CUSHING'S RESPONSE TO ↑ ICP

↓ Pulse rate
↓ Respiratory rate
↑ Pulse pressure
↑ Blood pressure

CAUSES OF ↓ GLASGOW COMA SCALE

Head Injury   Opiates/BZD
Alcohol   Poisons
Psychiatric   Infection
Uraemia   Ketosis
Epilepsy   Shock
Hypoxia

CAUSES OF CARPAL TUNNEL SYNDROME

Idiopathic   Menopause
Occupation   Pregnancy/OCP
Trauma   Hypothyroidism
Wrist fracture   Acromegaly
Ganglion   DM

Obesity   Amyloid
Lipoma   Gout
Alcoholism   Uraemia
TB   Rheumatoid arthritis

NERVE INJURY CLASSIFICATION

Neuropraxia (recovery hours/days):
    Disruption of conduction due to segment demyelination
    No wallerian degeneration
    Usually 2° blunt trauma/compression
Axonotmesis (recovery weeks/months):
    Disruption of axon with distal wallerian degeneration but an intact
    endoneurium
    Regrowth is at 1 mm/day
    Usually 2° blunt trauma/crush injury
Neurotmesis (often permanent):
    Disruption of nerve sheaths and axons, ie complete neurone
    disruption
    Proximal chromatolysis
    Limited regeneration without surgical intervention
    Usually 2° stab injury

FEATURES OF TIBIAL NERVE INJURIES

Paralysis of ankle and toe flexion with toe clawing
Shuffling gait (impaired take-off)
Muscle wasting of the sole
Loss of sensation of the sole
Flat foot (dysfunction of foot arches)

FEATURES OF PERONEAL NERVE INJURY

Paralysis of anterior and lateral compartment
Loss of dorsiflexion and toe extension (foot drop)
High stepping gait to clear ground
Normal-looking foot

REFLEXES

Biceps – C5/6
Brachioradialis – C6
Triceps – C7
Patella – L2/3
Achilles – S1/2
Babinski – UMN lesion

CHAPTER FOUR

Cardiovascular

Cardiovascular

RISK FACTORS FOR ATHEROMATOUS DISEASE

Age   ↑ TG/Cholesterol
Male   Fatty diet
Smoker   Obesity
Family history   Hypothyroidism
DM   Hypercoagulability
Hypertension   Stimulant abuse

FEATURES OF ACUTELY ISCHAEMIC LIMB

Paralysis   Pulseless
Paraesthesia   Pale
Painful   Perishingly cold

CAUSES OF POST-OPERATIVE HYPERTENSION

Pain   Pre-operative hypertension (see below)
Urinary retention   Inotropes
Hypercapnoea   Withdrawal of normal medication
Hypoxia

CAUSES OF HYPERTENSION

Essential (90%)

Renovascular: Chronic renal failure   Co-arctation of the aorta
                  Renal artery stenosis   Renin secreting tumours
                  Glomerular nephritis   Pre-eclampsia

Endocrine: Hyper/hypothyroidism   Acromegaly
                  Phaeochromocytoma   Conn's syndrome
                  Hyperparathyroidism   OCP
                  Cushing's syndrome

59

CAUSES OF ANEURYSMS

Age-related degeneration
Inflammatory
Congenital, eg Berry aneurysm
Connective tissue disease (Marfan's, Ehlers Danlos)

Atheroma
Traumatic
Syphilitic
Mycotic

COMPLICATIONS OF ANEURYSMAL DISEASE

Rupture
Embolism
Ischaemia

Thrombosis
Dissection
Pressure effects

COMPLICATIONS OF AORTIC SURGERY

Haemorrhage
Stroke
Myocardial infarction
Renal failure
Graft thrombosis
Graft infection
Distal embolism

Spinal ischaemia
Colonic ischaemia
DIC
ARDS
False aneurysm
Aorto-enteric fistula

CONGENITAL CARDIAC DEFECTS

R-L shunt (early cyanosis):

Tetralogy of Fallot
Transposition of the great vessels
Truncus arteriosus
Tricuspid atresia

L-R shunt (late cyanosis):

Ventricular septal defect
Atrial septal defect
Patent ductus arteriosus

TETRALOGY OF FALLOT

Pulmonary stenosis
Overriding aorta
Right ventricular hypertrophy
Ventricular septal defect

CAUSES OF ATRIAL FIBRILLATION (AF)

'Lone'
IHD
Mitral valve disease
Hyperthyroidism
Hypertension
Cardiomyopathy
Endocarditis
Constrictive pericarditis
Atrial myxoma
Hypoxia

Post-cardiac surgery
Pulmonary embolism
Alcohol excess
Haemachromatosis
Sarcoidosis
Lung CA
Pneumonia
Hypokalaemia
Hypomagnesaemia
Hypovolaemia

CAUSES OF NEUROPATHIC ULCERS

DM
Idiopathic
Vitamin B_{12} deficiency
Hypothyroidism
Alcohol
Amiodarone

HIV
TB
Leprosy
Syphilis
PRV
Malignancy

RAYNAUD'S SYNDROME

1°: Vasomotor – Raynaud's Dx
2°: Connective tissue Dx – SLE, PAN, RA, scleroderma, Sjörgen's syndrome
   Arterial Dx – artheroma, Buerger's Dx, thoracic outlet obstruction
   Trauma – frostbite, vibration
   Drugs – ergot, OCP, β-blockers

Haematological –   PRV, cryoglobulinaemia, cold agglutins, leukaemia, thrombocytosis, monoclonal gammaopathies

INDICATIONS FOR AMPUTATION

Peripheral vascular disease   Necrotising fasciitis
Trauma   Thromboangiitis obliterans
Malignancy   Burns
Osteomyelitis   Frostbite
Gas gangrene

COMPLICATIONS OF DM

Arterial disease: Atheroma/arteriosclerosis
                    Micro/macro-vascular dx

Skin disease: Carbuncle/furuncle   Necrobiosis lipoidica
                    Cellulitis   Impaired wound healing
                    Neuropathic ulceration

Renal disease: Glomerulonephritis   Papillary necrosis
                    Hypertension   Pyelonephritis/UTI
                    Renal artery stenosis

Eyes: Cataracts   Retinopathy
                    Infection

RISK FACTORS FOR DVT

Peri-operative: Trauma   MI
                  Immobility   CCF
                  Lower limb surgery

Patient: Age   Inherited thrombophilia
                                        (see below)
                  Obesity   Pregnancy/OCP
                  Previous Hx   Inflammatory bowel disease
                  Malignancy   Dysfibrinogenaemia
                  Nephrotic syndrome

CAUSES OF THROMBOSIS

Intimal damage:	Atheroma/arteriosclerosis	Instrumentation
	Inflammation	External compression
	Chemicals/toxins	Trauma

Altered blood flow: Turbulence – stenosis, anastomosis, prosthesis
Stasis – AF, pelvic mass, aneurysm

Altered blood: Platelets – ↑ no. of platelets or platelet activation
Coagulation – protein C and S deficiency, factor V Leiden, AT III deficiency, antiphospholipid syndrome
Cells – increased viscosity, dehydration, Waldenstrom's macroglobulinaemia, multiple myeloma, myeloproliferative disorders, ↑ viscosity, dehydration

DISSEMINATED INTRAVASCULAR COAGULATION (DIC)

Infection – septicaemia, aspergillosis, systemic candidiasis, malaria
Shock – trauma, burns, major surgery, pancreatitis
Vascular – cardiopulmonary bypass, severe vasculitis
Obstetric – septic abortion, abruption, eclampsia, amniotic embolism
Malignancy – metastatic CA (pancreas, lung, ovary, prostate)
Hepatic – cirrhosis, acute necrosis
Iatrogenic – ABO incompatibility, drug reaction

FEATURES OF PE

Dyspnoea/tachypnoea   ↑ JVP
Chest pain   Shock
Tachycardia   Prominent P2
Fever   Cyanosis
DVT   Hypoxia
Haemoptysis   Pleural rub
EMD

CARDIOVASCULAR

INHERITED THROMBOPHILIA

Factor V Leiden
Antithrombin III deficiency
Protein C deficiency
Protein S deficiency

PATHOGENESIS OF LIPODERMATOSCLEROSIS (THEORIES)

Venous stagnations – stagnant blood at increased pressure in veins causes ischaemia
Fibrin cuff – fibrin leaking from blood vessels acts as a barrier to oxygen and nutrition
White cell trapping – white cells that become trapped in the microcirculation cause tissue damage
Growth factor trapping – perpetuates local inflammation

COMPLICATIONS OF VARICOSE VEINS

Venous eczema	Venous pigmentation (haemosiderin)
Venous ulceration	Lipodermatosclerosis
Bleeding	Corona lebectasia
Oedema	Superficial thrombophlebitis

TRIBUTARIES OF THE LONG SAPHENOUS VEIN AT THE SAPHENOFEMORAL JUNCTION

Superior inferior epigastric	Superficial circumflex iliac
Deep external pudendal	Anterioro-lateral thigh
Superficial external pudendal	Postero-medial thigh

CAUSES OF ANKLE SWELLNG

Hypoproteinaemia	A-V malformation
Liver failure	DVT
Renal failure	Lipodystrophic disorder

CCF
Protein losing enteropathy
Fluid overload
Lymphoedema
Trauma

Parkes–Weber syndrome
Allergy
Hereditary angioedema
Immobility

LUMP IN POPLITEAL FOSSA

Lipoma
Sebaceous cyst
Bursitis
Baker's cyst

Saphena varix
DVT
Popliteal aneurysm
Neuroma

COMPLICATIONS OF TRANSFUSION

Immunological:	Immediate haemolysis	Delayed haemolysis
	Febrile reaction	Graft versus host disease
	Immunosuppression	TRALI
Technical:	Fluid overload	Air embolism
	Iron overload	Hypothermia
Metabolic:	Hypocalcaemia	Acid-base disturbance
	Hyperkalaemia	
Infective:	Bacterial – syphilis	
	Viral – Hep B+C, HIV, EBV, CMV, parvovirus	
	Parasitic – malaria	
	Prion – CJD?	
Haematological:	Coagulopathy	
	DIC	

ANAEMIA

Normocytic:	Haemorrhage
	Enzyme defect eg G6PDH, PK
	Membrane defect eg spherocytosis elliptosis
	Sickle cell disease
	Autoimmune haemolytic anaemia
	Bone marrow failure
	Anaemia of chronic disease
Macrocytic:	B_{12}/folate deficiency
	Antimetabolites
	Reticulocytosis
Microcytic:	Iron deficiency anaemia
	Thalassaemia
	Anaemia of chronic disease

CHAPTER FIVE

Endocrine and Breast

Endocrine and Breast

CAUSES OF SIADH

CNS disorders – infection, trauma, surgery, malignancy
Pulmonary disease – infection, trauma, surgery, malignancy
Ectopic ADH – SCLC, pancreas CA, prostate CA
Drugs – opioids, antiepileptics, sedatives, chemotherapy, antidepressants
Other – Guillian–Barré syndrome, pancreatitis, porphyria, alcohol withdrawal

MULTIPLE ENDOCRINE NEOPLASIA (MEN)

MEN I (AD – Werner syndrome, chromosome 11)
    Pituitary adenoma
    Pancreatic islet cell tumour
    Parathyroid hyperplasia/adenoma
    Adrenal cortex tumour

MEN IIa (AD – Sipple syndrome, chromosome 10)
    Medullary thyroid CA
    Phaeochromocytoma
    Parathyroid adenoma/hyperplasia

MEN III (or IIb – chromosome 10)
    Medullary thyroid CA
    Phaeochromocytoma
    Multiple mucosal neuromas

FEATURES OF PHAEOCHROMOCYTOMA

10% malignant   10% bilateral
10% extra-adrenal   10% paediatric
10% calcified   10% familial

CAUSES OF CUSHING'S SYNDROME

Pituitary tumour (Cushing's disease – 75%)
Adrenal tumour (15%)
Ectopic ACTH (NSCLC and carcinoid – 9%)
Ectopic CRH (rare)

FEATURES OF CUSHING'S SYNDROME

Truncal obesity   Weakness
Acne   Hypertension
Abdominal striae   Polyuria/dipsia
Kyphosis/Buffalo hump   Depression
Oedema   DM/glycosuria
Bruising   Osteoporosis
Hirsutism   Amenorrhoea
Moon facies   Hypokalaemia
Proximal myopathy

CAUSES OF ADDISON'S DISEASE

Idiopathic   Infection, eg TB, histoplasmosis, HIV
Autoimmune   Meningococcal septicaemia
Bilateral adrenalectomy 'Crisis' post-steroid withdrawal
Metastatic deposit   Metyrapone
Sarcoid   Ketoconazole
Amyloid

FEATURES OF ADDISON'S DISEASE

Pigmentation
Weight loss
Hypotension
Abdominal pain
Anaemia

Hyponatraemia
Hyperkalaemia
Hypercalcaemia
Hypoglycaemia

CAUSES OF HYPERTHYROIDISM

Graves' disease
Solitary toxic nodule
Toxic multinodular goitre
Iatrogenic (thyroxine, iodine)
De Quervain's thyroiditis

Post-partum
Thyroid CA
Ovarian teratoma
Ectopic thyroid

FEATURES OF HYPERTHYROIDISM

Heat intolerance
Weight loss
Diarrhoea
Anxiety
Tachycardia
Atrial fibrillation
Proximal myopathy
Acropathy

Fine tremor
Eye signs (see below)
Goitre
Sweating
Palmar erythema
Warm peripheries
Amenorrhoea

EYE SIGNS IN HYPERTHYROIDISM

Lid retraction
Lid lag
Peri-orbital oedema
Proptosis
Exophthalmos

Chemosis
Diploplia
Ophthalmoplegia
Corneal involvement
Optic nerve compression

FEATURES OF HYPOTHYROIDISM

Cold intolerance
Weight gain
Constipation
Tiredness
Bradycardia
Dry skin
IHD/CCF

Slow relaxing reflexes
Loss of outer third of eyebrow
Oedema
Sluggish mentation
Pre-tibial myxoedema
Menstrual irregularities

FEATURE OF ACROMEGALY

Coarse facies
Enlarged extremities
Enlarged jaw
Hyperhidrosis
Arthropathy
Renal calculi

Hypertension
DM
Carpal tunnel syndrome
LVH
IHD
Increased incidence of CRC

FUNCTIONS OF CALCIUM

Clotting
Conduction
Constituent of bone
Co-factor
Contraction

CAUSES OF HYPOCALCAEMIA

Hypoparathyroidism
Vitamin D deficiency
Malabsorption states
Chronic renal failure
Acute pancreatitis
Rhabdomyolysis

FEATURES OF HYPOCALCAEMIA

Paraesthesia
Fitting
Circumoral numbness
Cramps
Psychosis
Depression

Tetany, eg carpopedal/laryngospasm
ECG abnormalities
Dystonia
Chvostek's/Trousseau's sign
Cataracts (chronic)

CAUSES OF HYPERCALCAEMIA

Iatrogenic (thiazides, lithium)
Hyperparathyroidism
Milk alkali syndrome
Sarcoid
Vit D excess
Paget's disease
Dehydration
Immobility
TB

Addison's disease
Hyperthyroidism
Acromegaly
Lymphoma
Phaeochromocytoma
Bone mets. – breast, kidney, lung, thyroid, prostate
Multiple myeloma
Familial hypocalciuric hypercalcaemia

FEATURES OF HYPERCALCAEMIA

Abdominal pain
Weight loss
Constipation
Vomiting
Nausea/anorexia
Muscle weakness
Psychiatric disease

Polyuria
Polydipsia
Dehydration
Calculi
Renal failure
Arrhythmia
Cardiac arrest

CAUSES OF SODIUM ABNORMALITIES

	Hypovolaemia	Normovolaemic	Hypervolaemic
↓ Na$^+$	GI loss	SIADH	Cardiac failure
	Renal loss	Hypothyroidism	Hepatic failure
	Ketosis	Polydipsia	Renal failure
	Addison's syndrome		
↑ Na$^+$	GI loss	Diabetes inspidus	Hypertonic fluid
	Renal loss	Insensible loss	
	Osmotic diuresis	Conn's syndrome	
	Burns		

BREAST CA RISK FACTORS

Age
Nulliparity
Early menarche/late menopause
Family history
Previous history
BRCA gene carrier
Hormone replacement therapy
OCP
Smoking
Hyperplasia with atypia
Ionising radiation

BREAST EXAMINATION FINDINGS IN MALIGNANCY

Hard lump
Lump with irregular margins
Fixity of lump
Skin tethering
Palpable axillary nodes
Ulceration
Nipple change (see below)

NIPPLE CHANGE IN MALIGNANCY

Discoloration
Discharge
Depression
Deviation
Displacement
Destruction

HISTOLOGY OF INVASIVE BREAST CANCER

Ductal
Lobular
Medullary
Not otherwise specified

Papillary
Cribriform
Mucoid

BREAST CANCERS SUITABLE FOR CONSERVATION SURGERY

Single clinical/radiological lesion
Tumour less than 4 cm
No sign of locally advanced tumour
No sign of extensive nodal involvement
No sign of metastasis

CAUSES OF GYNAECOMASTIA

Physiological – neonates, puberty, old age
Antihypertensives – ACE inhibitors, spironolactone, calcium channel blockers
Antimicrobials – metronidazole, isoniazid, ketoconazole
Other drugs – cimetidine, digoxin, oestrogens, steroids
Illicit drugs – marijuana, amphetamine
Endocrine – hypo/hyperthyroidism, gonadal failure, acromegaly
Other – liver failure, testicular tumours, lymphoma, starvation, Klinefelter's/Kallman's syndrome

CHAPTER SIX
Plastics and ENT

Plastics and ENT

SKIN LESIONS

Benign:
- Keratoacanthoma
- Seborrhoeic wart
- Solar keratosis
- Keloid/hypertrophic scar
- Dermoid cyst
- Pyogenic granuloma
- Epidermal/sebaceous cyst
- Dermatofibroma/histiocytoma
- Benign pigmented naevi
- Squamous cell papilloma/skin tags
- Senile keratosis

Malignant:
- BCC
- Melanoma
- Paget's disease
- SCC
- Bowen's disease

BENIGN PIGMENTED NAEVI

Lentigo
Junctional naevus
Dermal naevus
Compound naevus
Blue naevus

TYPES OF MELANOMA

Lentigo maligna
Nodular
Amelanotic
Superficial spreading
Acral

RISK FACTORS FOR MELANOMA

Fair skin   Family history of dysplastic naevi
Redhead   Albinism
Celtic race   Xeroderma pigmentosa
Intermittent UVB light exposure

POOR PROGNOSIS IN MELANOMA

Male   Breslow > 0.75 mm
Trunk   Vascular invasion
Ulceration   Neural invasion
Regression   High mitotic rate

FEATURES OF MALIGNANCY IN MELANOMA

Change in size   Loss of surface markings
Change in colour   Ulceration/inflammation
Lymphadenopathy   Varied colour
Bleeding   Halo
Irregular border   Greater than 5 mm diameter
Satellite lesion

BURNS AS BODY SURFACE AREA

Head   9%   Legs   18%
Arms   9%   Front torso 18%
Groin 1%   Back torso   18%
(Palm 1%)

COMPLICATIONS OF BURNS

Death (fluid loss and infection)   Burn diabetes
Septicaemia   Hypercatabolic state
Hypovolaemia   Curling ulcer
Hyper/hyponatraemia   DIC
Compartment syndrome   ARDS
Circumferential burn (Eschar)   CO poisoning

CLOSURE OF A WOUND/DEFECT

Primary closure
Heal by secondary intention
Split-skin graft
Full-thickness graft

Random flap
Axial flap
Free flap

COMPLICATIONS OF TRACHEOSTOMY

Haemorrhage
Nerve injury
Vocal cord palsy
Pneumothorax
Pneumomediastinum
Subcutaneous emphysema
Cellulitis
Stenosis
Fistula

Displacement
Blockage
Pneumonia
Atelectasis
Aspiration
Asphyxia
Tracheomalacia
Cricoid injury
Dysphagia

CAUSES OF STRIDOR

Luminal:	TB	Foreign body
Mural:	Epiglottitis	Papilloma
	Croup	Motor neurone disease
	Malignancy	Recurrent laryngeal nerve palsy
	Granuloma	Angioneurotic oedema
	Haemangioma	Laryngomalacia
Extra-mural:	Goitre	Post-neck surgery
	Mediastinal tumour	Trauma
	Lymphadenopathy	

PLASTICS AND ENT

CAUSES OF PAROTID SWELLING

Unilateral: Benign tumour   Acute parotiditis
              Malignant tumour   Lymphadenopathy
              Calculus   Facial nerve neuroma
              Sialadenitis

Bilateral: Alcohol   Acromegaly
              Malnutrition   DM
              Pancreatitis   Sjörgen's syndrome
              Mumps   Lymphoma
              Sarcoid   Leukaemia
              Cirrhosis   Amyloid
              Cystic fibrosis   Hyperlipidaemia

SALIVARY TUMOURS

Of which 80% are parotid
Of which 80% are benign
Of which 80% are pleomorphic adenoma
50% minor gland tumours are malignant
33% submandibular tumours are malignant

HISTOLOGY OF SALIVARY TUMOURS

Benign: Pleomorphic adenoma   Duct papilloma
             Adenolymphoma (Warthin's)   Papillary cystadenoma
             Myoepithelial adenoma

Malignant: Adenoid cystic CA   Adeno CA
             SCC   Undifferentiated CA

CAUSES OF FACIAL NERVE PALSY

Bell's/idiopathic (40%)

Intracranial: Tumour   Cholesteatoma
                CVA   Meningitis
                MS   Polio

Extracranial: Otitis media   Surgery
                Ramsey–Hunt syndrome   Tumour
                Trauma/fracture   Guillian–Barré syndrome

FEATURES OF MALIGNANCY IN PAROTID TUMOURS

VII nerve involvement   Hard
Rapid growth   Fixed
Pain   Irregular surface/edge
Hyperaemic

COMPLICATION OF PAROTID SURGERY

VII nerve injury   Salivary fistula
Great auricular nerve injury   Gustatory sweating (Frey's syndrome)
Wound infection   Wound dimple
Haemorrhage

EMBRYOLOGICAL PHARYNGEAL POUCHES

1st – Middle ear, eustachian tube and mastoid air cells
2nd – Palatine tonsil
3rd – Inferior parathyroids and thymus
4th – Superior parathyroids
5th – Parafollicular C cells

CAUSES OF THYROID SWELLING

Solitary: Solitary cyst   CA
          Haemorrhage into a cyst   Adenoma
          Multinodular goitre
Diffuse: Multinodular goitre   Physiological
          Hashimoto's thyroiditis   CA
          Graves' disease   Iodine deficiency/endemic goitre

HISTOLOGY OF MALIGNANT THYROID TUMOURS

Papillary –   least aggressive with LN spread
Follicular –   moderately aggressive with vascular spread
Anaplastic –   aggressive with very poor prognosis
Medullary –   from calcitonin secreting parafollicular C cells
Lymphoma –   particularly in Hashimoto's thyroiditis

INDICATIONS FOR THYROID SURGERY

Failed medical treatment
Compression
Carcinoma
Cosmesis

COMPLICATIONS OF THYROIDECTOMY

Haematoma
Respiratory obstruction
Recurrent laryngeal nerve injury
Superior laryngeal nerve injury
Keloid/hyperplastic scar

Hypothyroidism
Hypoparathyroidism
Hypocalcaemia (early and late)
Thyroid storm/crisis

CHAPTER SEVEN
Your Lists

Your Lists

Bibliography

Andrews S. *MRCS Core Modules: Essential Revision Notes*, 2nd edition, PasTest Limited, 2002

Aird I, Burnard KG, Young AE. *The New Aird's Companion in Surgical Studies*, 2nd edition, Churchill Livingstone, 1997

Appleby AG, Solomon L. *Concise System of Orthopaedics and Fractures*, 2nd edition, Butterworth Heinemann, 1994

Chan CLH, Hart AJ. *Viva Practice for Intercollegiate MRCS (Part 3)*, PasTest Limited, 2004

Ellis H. *Clinical Anatomy – A Revision and Applied Anatomy for Clinical Students*, Blackwell Science, 2002

Esser M, McRae M. *Practical Fracture Treatment*, 4th edition, Churchill Livingstone, 2002

Kirk RM, Ribbins WJ. *Clinical Surgery in General: RCS Course Manual*, Churchill Livingstone, 2003

Surgery – The Continuously Updated Resource of Surgery, The Medicine Publishing Company Limited (continuously revised)

STEP – Surgeons in Training Education Programme, Royal College of Surgeons

Parchment Smith C, Hernon C. *MRCS Systems Modules: Essential Revision Notes*, 2nd edition, PasTest Limited, 2000

Parchment Smith C. *Surgical Short Cases for the MRCS Clinical Examination*, PasTest Limited, 2002

Index

INDEX